Insulin Resistance Eating Plan

A Beginner's 2-Week Step-by-Step Guide for Women to Manage PCOS and Prediabetes, With Sample Curated Recipes

mf

copyright © 2021 Mary Golanna

All rights reserved No part of this book may be reproduced, or stored in a retrieval system, or transmitted in any form or by any means, electronic, mechanical, photocopying, recording, or otherwise, without express written permission of the publisher.

Disclaimer

By reading this disclaimer, you are accepting the terms of the disclaimer in full. If you disagree with this disclaimer, please do not read the guide.

All of the content within this guide is provided for informational and educational purposes only, and should not be accepted as independent medical or other professional advice. The author is not a doctor, physician, nurse, mental health provider, or registered nutritionist/dietician. Therefore, using and reading this guide does not establish any form of a physician-patient relationship.

Always consult with a physician or another qualified health provider with any issues or questions you might have regarding any sort of medical condition. Do not ever disregard any qualified professional medical advice or delay seeking that advice because of anything you have read in this guide. The information in this guide is not intended to be any sort of medical advice and should not be used in lieu of any medical advice by a licensed and qualified medical professional.

The information in this guide has been compiled from a variety of known sources. However, the author cannot attest to or guarantee the accuracy of each source and thus should not be held liable for any errors or omissions.

You acknowledge that the publisher of this guide will not be held liable for any loss or damage of any kind incurred as a result of this guide or the reliance on any information provided within this guide. You acknowledge and agree that you assume all risk and responsibility for any action you undertake in response to the information in this guide.

Using this guide does not guarantee any particular result (e.g., weight loss or a cure). By reading this guide, you acknowledge that there are no guarantees to any specific outcome or results you can expect.

All product names, diet plans, or names used in this guide are for identification purposes only and are the property of their respective owners. The use of these names does not imply endorsement. All other trademarks cited herein are the property of their respective owners.

Where applicable, this guide is not intended to be a substitute for the original work of this diet plan and is, at most, a supplement to the original work for this diet plan and never a direct substitute. This guide is a personal expression of the facts of that diet plan.

Where applicable, persons shown in the cover images are stock photography models and the publisher has obtained the rights to use the images through license agreements with third-party stock image companies.

Table of Contents

Introduction	7
What Is Insulin Resistance?	9
Causes of Insulin Resistance	10
Symptoms	10
Complications	11
Diagnosis and Tests	11
Insulin Resistance and Diabetes	12
How Insulin Resistance Develops to Type 2 Diabetes	13
Insulin Resistance in Women	13
Conquering Insulin Resistance	16
Make a Plan	16
Exercise	16
Adopt a Healthy Diet	17
Medical Treatment and Medication	18
A Two-Week Self-Treatment Plan	19
Samples of a Healthy Diet	23
Arugula and Mushroom Salad	24
Honey Chicken and Avocado Salad	25
Chicken Salad	27
Egg Salad with Avocados	28
Vegetable Broth	29
Tahini Salmon	31
Baked Flounder	33
Baked Salmon	34
Pine Nut Quinoa Bowl	35
Spinach and Chickpeas	37
Roasted Veggies	38
Mixed Vegetable Roast with Lemon Zest	39
Spinach Berry Lemon Smoothie	40

Keto Zucchini Walnut Bread	41
Zero Carb Buttery Noodles	43
Tangy Lemon Fish	44
Salad Medley	46
Conclusion	**48**
References and Helpful Links	**49**

Introduction

You can conquer Insulin Resistance!

Insulin Resistance is a hazardous condition that robs you of a healthy and happy life. Usually, insulin-resistant people are also in the prediabetes stage, which is a step away from the debilitating disease of diabetes. Prediabetes indicates that your blood glucose points are higher than normal but not high enough to be established as diabetes.

In the United States alone, 84 million people suffer from prediabetes—that is about 1 in 3 American adults. About 90% of them are unaware that they are insulin-resistant or have prediabetes. It is also known that females are more likely affected by insulin resistance as compared to males.

Insulin resistance happens when cells in your body and major organs don't react well to insulin and can't take up glucose from your blood. Consequently, the pancreas produces more insulin to help your cells absorb glucose. Generally, your blood glucose levels will stay in a good, healthy range as long as your pancreas produces enough insulin to strengthen your cells' response to insulin.

Prediabetes or insulin resistance happens when your blood glucose levels are elevated than normal but not high enough to be diagnosed as diabetes. If there is not enough insulin in your system, extra glucose will remain in your bloodstream instead of being absorbed by your cells.

In this guide, you will discover:

- The nature of Insulin Resistance
- Causes and symptoms of this condition
- The relation between Diabetes and Insulin Resistance
- The lifestyle changes to conquer Insulin Resistance
- Samples of a healthy diet to cure Insulin Resistance

However, do not fret. Insulin resistance can be reversed by following this guide so that you may avoid diabetes and other major diseases in your life.

What Is Insulin Resistance?

Insulin resistance happens when cells in your liver, fat, and muscles don't respond well to insulin and can't process glucose from the blood for energy.

Insulin is a hormone produced by your pancreas that allows your body to process glucose for energy. Glucose is a type of sugar usually found in carbohydrates. The digestive system breaks down carbohydrates and transforms them into glucose—essentially a type of sugar that your body uses for energy. It is also called blood sugar, as it travels through your bloodstream into your cells.

People with diabetes have alleviated levels of glucose in their blood. They may not have enough insulin to move it through or their cells don't respond to insulin properly.

Studies also show that females are more likely to be insulin resistant than males, which requires proper medical attention particularly because of its risks that usually result in other medical conditions.

Causes of Insulin Resistance

There are numerous possible causes of insulin resistance. They include obesity, a dysfunctional pancreas, high blood pressure, abnormal cholesterol levels, pregnancy, hypoglycemia, obesity, chronic liver disease, and many others.

A family history of type 2 diabetes is also a major factor that leads to insulin resistance. People who are also 45 years or older, belonging to certain ethnic groups like Alaska Native, Asian American, Latino, African American, and others are prone to this condition.

In addition, certain medications also cause insulin resistance such as antimalarials, lithium, beta-blockers, and others.

Lastly, a bad lifestyle such as having an improper diet, lack of exercise, and being overweight leads to this disease.

Symptoms

- Dizziness, depression, constant feeling of tiredness
- Obesity and a waistline above 40 inches in men and 35 inches in women
- Recurrent urinary tract infection
- Patches of dark, velvety skin
- A HDL cholesterol level under 40 mg/dL in men and 50 mg/dL in women
- A fasting glucose level over 100 mg/dL

- A fasting triglyceride level over 150 mg/dL
- Blood pressure of 130/80 or higher

Complications

- Heart attack
- Severe high blood sugar
- Cancer and other malignancies
- Alzheimer's disease
- Stroke
- Kidney disease
- Eye problems
- Very low blood sugar

Diagnosis and Tests

Your physician will undergo these steps:

- Interview for your symptoms, sickness background, family medical history
- Physical Exam
- Oral glucose tolerance test (average sugar level)
- Hemoglobin A1c test (average blood glucose level)

Insulin Resistance and Diabetes

Diabetes happens when your body doesn't utilize insulin properly or doesn't produce the right amount of insulin. A study concluded that people with prediabetes or insulin resistance are up to 50% more likely to contract diabetes in the next 5 to 10 years. There are two types of diabetes.

Type 1 is an autoimmune disease that causes your own body to assault itself. Your body can't produce insulin because your immune system has destroyed all the cells in your pancreas that produce insulin.

Type 2 diabetes is the more common condition. Your body becomes more resistant to the effects of insulin. You need more insulin to achieve the same and right effects. Thus, your body overproduces more insulin to maintain your blood glucose levels to normal.

After many years of the overproduction of insulin, the insulin-producing cells in the pancreas are affected and burn out.

How Insulin Resistance Develops to Type 2 Diabetes

When you are insulin resistant, your pancreas produces extra insulin to make up for the deficiency. For a time, this will work out well and your blood sugar levels will be normal.

However, after some time, the pancreas won't be able to keep up. If you don't address this situation early enough through diet, exercise, and lifestyle changes your blood sugar levels will rise until you have prediabetes.

You will be diagnosed with type 2 diabetes when your fasting plasma glucose test results in 126 or higher, oral glucose tolerance reaches 200 or higher after the second test, and your A1c reaches 6.5% or above.

Insulin Resistance in Women

Insulin resistance affects more women than men. In some cases, women who have insulin resistance do not develop the general symptoms and conditions of the disease but have a higher risk of developing them.

Women with insulin resistance are also susceptible to many diverse complications when they are pregnant. Women are more likely to have irregular menstrual cycles. This means that they could experience having light periods or even no periods at all.

Women with insulin resistance are also at a higher risk of hypoglycemia during pregnancy. This means a low blood sugar level.

As such, there is a strong possibility that the body will not process and utilize glucose properly. This can result in dangerous dehydration and low blood glucose levels.

Women with insulin resistance also are at an elevated risk of developing PCOS (Polycystic Ovary Syndrome), where the woman's chances of having ovarian cysts become high.

PCOS is a common cause of female infertility. Symptoms include irregular periods, thinning scalp hair, acne, and excessive hair growth on the body and face. According to the Centers for Disease and Control (CDC), 50% of women with PCOS develop Type 2 diabetes.

PCOS usually happens during menopause when her hormones become imbalanced. Thus, the levels of insulin and other female hormones tend to increase, which can result in obesity. The imbalance also causes cysts to grow and increase in the ovaries. This means that these cysts are likely to grow big enough and develop into a tumors.

Women who are insulin-resistant are also prone to developing hypertension. High blood pressure is marked by the presence of too much fluid in the blood. High blood sugar levels residing in the blood are the effect of insulin resistance.

The kidneys of insulin-resistant women also wrestle with the continuous attempts to remove excess fluid from the body. The kidneys can be inflamed and eventually become damaged. This impairment of the kidneys can result in fluid build-up in the blood and result in numerous medical conditions.

Finally, urinary tract infections (UTIs) can result when bacteria enter the urinary tract, including the kidney, bladder, and urethra. UTI is much more prevalent in women than in men. UTI also happens more to people with diabetes because the sugar in the urine becomes a breeding ground for the growth of bacteria.

Conquering Insulin Resistance

Make a Plan

A well-prepared plan is a cornerstone of a successful program to combat Insulin Resistance. You should solicit the help of physicians, professionals, family, and friends to support you in your goals and lifestyle changes. With the right attitude and a firm determination, you can conquer this dangerous condition.

Exercise

Lack of exercise and physical inactivity has been directly linked to insulin resistance. Physical movement and exercise make you more sensitive to insulin, which makes the right absorption of glucose.

Adequate exercise also leads to weight loss and good general health like avoiding high sugar levels, reduction of stress, and getting better sleep.

The Diabetes Prevention Program of the National Institutes of Health revealed that losing five to seven percent of a person's weight greatly reduces the chances of contracting diabetes.

Adopt a Healthy Diet

Setting a proper diet plan is key to managing insulin resistance. An insulin-resistance diet is one of the most significant weight loss programs that you adopt in managing your condition.

You don't need special or expensive foods to take for an insulin-resistance diet. It takes patience and determination to adopt such a diet, because you may be eating foods that you are not accustomed to eating.

You should include in your daily diet food that contains more healthy carbohydrates such as fruits, legumes, and vegetables. Lean meat, fish, and chicken should also be included in your list. Eat also three times a day, instead of having more meals in the day.

In general, you should also avoid foods that contain too much sugar or starch.

Key points of a healthy diet:

- *Aim for the right weight.* Ask your doctor or nutritionist how much you should weigh for your weight goal
- *Adopt healthy habits.* Don't attempt to do a crash diet. This can be dangerous. Having a new meal plan requires patience and determination as you will change your diet— a departure from the food that you used to

eat. For example, you should forgo your favorite soda drink.
- *Don't skip meals.* Often people think that by skipping meals, you take fewer calories and lose weight. On the contrary, skipping meals makes your insulin and blood sugar levels erratic. This can lead to more belly fat and make you more resistant to insulin.
- *Focus on food quality and calories.* There are many views on the right mix of protein, carbs, and fats. Keep watch on your total calories consumed. For example, skip the white rice in favor of whole grains.

Medical Treatment and Medication

Having the right doctor to diagnose and treat insulin resistance is key in managing this disease.

You should set a regular check-up routine with your physician to monitor your progress and glucose levels. Medications that your doctor would prescribe to you include metformin (Glucophage, Foretamet, Riomet, and the like) to aid in stabilizing your blood sugar level.

If your blood glucose levels are not managed well because of medication, diet, exercise, and lifestyle changes, insulin injections may be called for. If insulin resistance is already progressing into diabetes, your doctor may introduce you to insulin injections. They act as a supplement or replacement to the insulin in your body.

A Two-Week Self-Treatment Plan

Diagnosis Stage

Day 1- 2

Have regular check-ups with your doctor, including all the diagnostic tests. You should also see your physician as soon as possible if you experience dizziness, fatigue, general body weakness, and other negative physical signs.

Preparing Your Diet Plan

Day 3-5

Based on your actual condition and with the recommendation of your doctor, you should formulate your appropriate diet plan. Enumerate the right menus and recipes that would be palatable to you. List down the ingredients and formulate a shopping list.

As you progress in your diet list, update your plan according to the state of your insulin resistance condition.

Generally, these are the types of food that you should consider in your diet plan:

- *Vegetables*. Dark green, leafy, fresh vegetables like spinach are low in carbohydrates and calories. Packed with nutrients, you can take them as much as you want. Canned or frozen veggies should have no added salt, fat, and sugar.
- *Fruits*. These are great food choices because they are full of vitamins, fiber, and minerals. Avoid fruits in a can with syrup added.
- *Limited carbohydrates*. Cut down or limit your carbs. . Consume carbs in veggies, fruits, beans, whole grains, and low-fat dairy instead of processed foods such as pasta and white bread. Choose oats over toast for breakfast.
- *Fish*. Sardines, salmon, tuna, and other low-fat fish are good for alleviating insulin resistance.
- *High-fiber foods*. Taking more than fifty grams of fiber a day helps balance your blood sugar level. Examples are broccoli black beans, almonds, oatmeal, and lentils,
- *Low-fat dairy*. Low-fat milk and plain yogurt without fat give you protein, calcium, and fewer calories. In general, these foods lower insulin resistance.
- *Lean protein*. Eat enough protein not loaded with fat. Limit your intake of pork, beef, lamb, and chicken without the skin.

The types of food that you should avoid or limit:

- *Trans fats and saturated food.* These substances boost insulin resistance. They come from animal sources, such as fried foods, cheese, and other meats.
- *Sweetened beverages.* These drinks make you gain weight. They include soda drinks, iced tea, fruit drinks, iced teas, and the like.
- *Processed foods.* These types of food are not only harmful to insulin-resistant people but all people in general. Processed foods often have added salt, fat, and sugar.

Planning Your Exercise Routine

Day 6-7

Determine what is the suitable exercise according to your lifestyle. You should also consult your doctor about your determined exercise plan and routine.

Regular exercise makes your insulin more effective; making your body cells utilize glucose more effectively.

At least 30 minutes a day of moderate exercise five or more days a week is a good minimum target plan. This includes aerobic exercises like brisk walking, swimming, dancing, and the like. Consider also strength training and flexibility training.

Setting a Good Outlook in Life

Day 8-14

Conquering insulin resistance does not only involve diet management and exercise. It also includes having the right attitude and emotional outlook in life. Negativity produces hormones that adversely affect our organs and body in general.

- Have a positive outlook on life.
- Be joyful.
- Avoid too much stress.
- Manage anxiety and other life problems.

Samples of a Healthy Diet

Arugula and Mushroom Salad

Ingredients:

- 5 oz. arugula washed
- 1 lb. fresh mushrooms
- 1/4 teaspoon shoyu
- 1/2 red onion
- 1 tbsp. olive oil
- 1 tbsp. mirin

To make tofu cheese:

- 1/8 cup umeboshi vinegar
- 1/2 firm tofu

Instructions:

1. In a bowl, add the rinsed tofu. Crumble and pour in vinegar.
2. In a separate bowl add shoyu, red onions, salt, olive oil, and mirin. Mix to combine.
3. Add in the arugula and toss to combine with the dressing.
4. Serve and enjoy.

Honey Chicken and Avocado Salad

Ingredients:

- 4 chicken thighs, boneless
- 1/2 cup cherry tomatoes, halved
- 1/2 red onion, thinly sliced
- 1 head romaine lettuce, chopped
- 2 avocados, chopped

Marinade:

- 1 tbsp. olive oil
- 1 tsp. salt
- 2 cloves garlic, minced
- 1 jalapeño pepper, minced
- 1/2 tsp. chili powder
- 1 tbsp. honey
- 4 tbsp. lime juice

Dressing:

- 1 tsp. salt
- 4 tbsp. olive oil
- 1/2 tsp. pepper
- 2 tbsp. honey
- 4 tbsp. lime juice

Instructions:

1. Combine all the chicken marinade ingredients in a container.
2. Add in the thighs and allow to marinate for an hour at least.
3. Cook chicken in a cast-iron skillet on high heat for about 4 minutes on each side.
4. In a large salad bowl, put in avocados, lettuce, red onion, and tomatoes.
5. Slice or shred the chicken before adding to the salad bowl.
6. In a separate bowl, combine the dressing ingredients and mix well.
7. While tossing the salad, add in the dressing.
8. Serve immediately.

Chicken Salad

Ingredients:

- 1 small can premium chunk chicken breast packed in water
- 1 stalk celery, large, finely chopped
- 1/4 cup reduced-fat mayonnaise
- 4 romaine leaves or red leaf lettuce, washed and trimmed
- 2 oz. blue cheese, crumbled
- 8 pcs. cherry tomatoes or 1 ripe tomato, quartered
- 1 cucumber, small and sliced thinly

Instructions:

1. Drain canned chicken and transfer to a bowl.
2. Put in celery and mayonnaise.
3. Mix lightly. Don't crush the chicken.
4. In a separate shallow bowl, place the lettuce neatly.
5. Add in the chicken salad in the middle and sprinkle blue cheese over it.
6. Add in tomatoes and cucumber slices around the plate.
7. Refrigerate before serving, cover with plastic wrap.

Egg Salad with Avocados

Ingredients:

- 3 medium-sized avocados
- 6 eggs, large and hard-boiled
- 1/3 red onion, medium size
- 3 celery ribs
- 4 tbsps. Mayonnaise
- 2 tbsps. Freshly squeezed lime juice
- 2 tsp. brown mustard
- 1/2 tsp. cumin powder
- 1 tsp. hot sauce
- Salt and pepper

Instructions:

1. Chop the eggs, celery, and onion.
2. Set aside the avocados, then combine the rest of the ingredients.
3. Slice avocado in half to take out the pit.
4. Stuff the avocado by spooning the egg salad on its cave.
5. Serve and enjoy.

Vegetable Broth

Ingredients:

- 1 tbsp. oil
- 2 leeks, sliced
- 2 carrots, sliced
- 2 ribs celery
- ¼ tsp. salt
- 8 cups water

To make the soup:

- 1 tbsp. oil
- 2 cups potatoes, diced
- 1 cup mushrooms, diced
- 1.5 cups cauliflower, diced
- 1 cup onion, diced
- 1 cup celery, diced
- 1 cup carrot, diced
- 1.5 cups red beans, cooked
- 2 sprigs rosemary
- 4 sprigs thyme
- 2 cups spinach

Instructions:

1. To a pot on medium heat, add oil and leeks.
2. Cook for about three minutes or until they start to soften up.

3. Add carrots and top of a few celery stalks with leaves.
4. Cover with water.
5. Add salt. Bring to a simmer and cook until carrots are very tender but not mushy.
6. Turn off the heat and let it cool down a little.
7. When the broth has cooled down, strain out the veggies.
8. Remove carrots and set them aside.
9. Squeeze most of the liquid out of the leeks and celery.

To cook the soup:

1. Add carrots to some of the broth and blend.
2. With a pot on medium heat, add oil, onions, raw carrots, and celery. Cook until onions are translucent, approximately 3 to 5 minutes.
3. Add broth, potatoes, and herbs.
4. Bring to a simmer and cook for 10 minutes.
5. Add cauliflower and red beans.
6. Simmer for another 5 minutes.
7. Add the package of frozen green beans and cook until the potatoes and cauliflower are tender, approximately for another 5 minutes.
8. At the end of cooking, add spinach.

Tahini Salmon

Instructions:

- 1/4 cup tahini
- 3 tbsp. fresh lemon juice
- 1 tsp. mashed garlic
- 1/4 tsp. salt
- 1/2 cup finely chopped cilantro
- 2 tbsp. roughly chopped toasted walnuts
- 2 tbsp. roughly chopped toasted almonds
- 1 tbsp. finely chopped onion
- 1 tsp. extra-virgin olive oil
- Pinch of cayenne, or to taste
- Freshly ground black pepper to taste
- 1 lb. wild salmon skin removed, fresh or frozen

Instructions:

1. In a bowl, combine the tahini, 2 tbsp. of lemon juice, 3 tbsp. of water, mashed garlic, and 1/8 tsp. of salt; set aside
2. In a separate bowl, combine the cilantro, walnuts, almonds, onion, olive oil, cayenne, black pepper, and 1/8 tsp. of salt.
3. Fill the bottom of a steamer with water and bring to a boil.
4. Season fish with 1 tbsp. of lemon juice.

5. Place it on a plate and put it on the top of the steamer. Cover and cook, taking care to remove while the fish is still pink inside, about 3 to 4 minutes.
6. Remove the fish from the steamer, top with the tahini mixture, and then with the cilantro mixture.
7. Serve warm or at room temperature.

Baked Flounder

Ingredients:

- 1 lb. flounder fillet
- 1 tbsp. extra-virgin olive oil
- 1/4 tsp. salt
- Freshly ground black pepper to taste
- 1 cup halved red grapes
- 1 cup chopped and toasted almonds
- 2 tbsp. finely chopped parsley
- 1 tbsp. lemon juice

Instructions:

1. Preheat the oven to 375°F. Place fish on a sheet tray and season with 1-1/2 tsp. of olive oil, 1/8 tsp of salt, and freshly ground black pepper.
2. In a bowl, combine the grapes, almonds, parsley, lemon juice, 1-1/2 tsp. of olive oil, 1/8 tsp of salt, and black pepper.
3. Place the fish in the oven and bake for 3 minutes, flip the fish, return to the oven until the fish is just beginning to flake but the center is still translucent for approximately 3 minutes. Take care not to overcook
4. Remove from the oven and serve immediately, topped with the grape mixture.

Baked Salmon

Ingredients:

- 2 salmon fillets
- 6 cups of fresh spinach
- 2 tsp. coconut oil
- 1 tsp. coconut oil
- 1/4 tsp. garlic powder
- 1/4 tsp. turmeric
- 3 large cloves of garlic
- lemon juice
- salt and pepper, to taste

Instructions:

1. Preheat the oven to 400℉.
2. Line a baking dish with parchment paper.
3. Marinate salmon fillets in lemon juice, coconut oil, garlic powder, turmeric, salt, and pepper.
4. Let it sit for a few minutes. This may also be done the night before to help the juices and flavor get into the salmon.
5. Once the oven is ready, bake salmon for 15 minutes.
6. Cook some of the garlic in a pan with coconut oil.
7. Add spinach and cook until ready. Season with salt and pepper to taste.
8. Take salmon out of the oven and put spinach beside.
9. Serve and enjoy.

Pine Nut Quinoa Bowl

Ingredients:

- 1 cup dry white quinoa, rinsed

Marinara sauce:

- 1/4 cup extra-virgin olive oil, preferably cold-pressed
- 2 tbsp. lemon juice
- 1-1/4 tbsp. agave nectar
- 2 cups sun-dried tomatoes, soaked in water for 2 hours
- 1 cup soaking water used for tomatoes
- 2 large Roma or heirloom tomatoes, diced
- 1/2 yellow onion, chopped
- 3-4 cloves garlic, crushed
- 1 handful fresh basil leaves, reserve some for garnish
- 2 tsp. dried oregano
- 1 tsp. sea salt
- A pinch of hot pepper flakes
- 1/4 cup pine nuts, reserve some for garnish

Instructions:

For the quinoa:

1. Combine rinsed quinoa with 2 cups of filtered water in a medium saucepan.
2. Bring to a full boil.
3. Reduce heat to low and let it simmer.

4. Cover the pan and cook until all the water is absorbed and the quinoa is fluffy and tender, for 15 to 20 minutes.

For the marinara sauce:

1. Add olive oil, lemon juice, agave nectar to a high-speed blender.
2. Add sun-dried tomatoes, Roma tomatoes, onions, garlic, basil, oregano, salt, and hot pepper flakes to the blender.
3. Blend until smooth, about 30 to 45 seconds. Use a tamper if necessary to support the proper blending of sauce.
4. If necessary, add additional tomato soaking water to thin sauce. This is ready to serve.
5. Optional: Set the sauce to simmer at a low temperature in a medium saucepan for 25 to 30 minutes.
6. Spoon the marinara sauce over the cooked quinoa in a serving bowl.
7. Top with pine nuts and fresh basil leaves.
8. Serve immediately.

Spinach and Chickpeas

Ingredients:

- 3 tbsp. extra virgin olive oil
- 1 onion, thinly sliced
- 4 cloves garlic, minced
- 1 tbsp. grated ginger
- ½ container grape tomatoes
- 1 lemon, zested and freshly juiced
- 1 tsp. crushed red pepper flakes
- 1 large can of chickpeas
- 6 cups spinach
- Sea salt to taste

Instructions:

1. Add extra virgin olive oil to a large skillet, add onion, and cook until the onion starts to brown.
2. Add garlic, ginger, tomatoes, lemon zest, red pepper flakes, and spinach. Cook for about 3 to 4 minutes.
3. Add cooked chickpeas and stir. Add oil if necessary.
4. Serve and enjoy.

Roasted Veggies

Ingredients:

- 1/2 lb. turnips
- 1/2 lb. carrots
- 1/2 lb. parsnips
- 2 shallots, peeled
- 1/4 tsp. ground black pepper
- 1 tbsps. extra-virgin olive oil
- 6 cloves garlic
- 3/4 tsp. kosher salt
- 2 tbsp. fresh rosemary needles

Instructions:

1. First, cut vegetables into bite-sized pieces.
2. Set the oven to 400°F.
3. Mix all the ingredients in a baking dish.
4. Roast the vegetables for 25 minutes until brown and tender.
5. Toss and roast again for 20- 25 minutes.
6. Serve and enjoy while hot.

Mixed Vegetable Roast with Lemon Zest

Ingredients:

- 1-1/2 cups broccoli florets
- 1-1/2 cups cauliflower florets
- 3/4 cup red bell pepper, diced
- 3/4 cup zucchini, diced
- 2 thinly sliced cloves of garlic
- 2 tsp. lemon zest
- 1 tbsp. olive oil
- A pinch of salt
- 1 tsp. dried and crushed oregano

Instructions:

1. Preheat the oven, set to 425°F.
2. Combine garlic and both florets in a baking pan. Drizzle oil over the vegetables and sprinkle with salt and oregano; stir long enough to coat. Roast for 10 minutes.
3. Add zucchini and bell pepper to the rest of the mix in the pan; toss to combine.
4. Continue roasting until the pieces are lightly browned and are crisp-tender.
5. Before serving, drizzle lemon zest over the vegetables and toss.
6. Enjoy while hot.

Spinach Berry Lemon Smoothie

Ingredients:

- 2 cups of fresh spinach leaves, rinsed and roughly chopped
- 1 frozen banana, sliced
- 7–8 frozen strawberries
- 1 tbsp. chia seeds
- 1 tbsp. lemon juice
- 2–3 cups of chilled coconut water

Instructions:

1. Add the spinach leaves to the blender.
2. Add frozen banana to the blender.
3. Add in the frozen strawberries, chia seeds, lemon juice, and coconut water.
4. Blend until all the ingredients combine well.

Keto Zucchini Walnut Bread

Ingredients:

- 3 large eggs
- 1/2 cup virgin olive oil
- 1 tsp. vanilla extract
- 2-1/4 cups fine almond flour
- 1-1/2 cups sweetener, erythritol
- 1/2 tsp. salt
- 1-1/2 tsp. baking powder
- 1/2 tsp. nutmeg, ground
- 1 tsp. cinnamon, ground
- 1/4 tsp. ginger, ground
- 1 cup zucchini, grated
- 1/2 cup walnuts, chopped

Instructions:

1. Preheat your oven to 350°F.
2. Whisk together the eggs, oil, and vanilla extract. Set aside.
3. Using another bowl, combine the baking powder, sweetener, almond flour, salt, cinnamon, nutmeg, and ginger powder. Set aside.
4. Squeeze the excess water from the zucchini using a paper towel or a cheesecloth.
5. Pour the zucchini into the egg mixture and whisk.

6. Add the flour mixture slowly into the egg and zucchini mixture. Blend using an electric blender until the mixture turns smooth.
7. Spray a loaf pan with avocado oil or baking spray.
8. Pour the zucchini batter into the loaf pan and smoothen the top evenly.
9. Spoon the chopped walnuts on top of the batter, lightly pressing the walnuts with the back of a spoon to press into the batter.
10. Pop the loaf pan into the oven and then bake for 60-70 minutes, or until the walnuts turn brown.
11. Cool in a cooling rack before slicing and serving.

Zero Carb Buttery Noodles

Ingredients:

- 7 oz. shirataki noodles
- 2 tbsp. unsalted butter
- 1 tbsp. grated parmesan
- salt
- black pepper
- fresh basil or parsley

Instructions:

1. Drain and rinse the noodles in cold water.
2. Transfer them to a bowl, and cover with boiling water for 5 minutes.
3. Drain again.
4. In a skillet, melt the butter over medium heat.
5. Add the noodles, and sprinkle in some salt.
6. Sauté for 3-4 minutes until the butter has been absorbed.
7. Add pepper to the task, garnish with parmesan and basil or parsley.

Tangy Lemon Fish

Ingredients:

- 200 g. Gurnard fresh fish fillets
- 3 tbsp. butter
- 1 tbsp. fresh lemon juice
- 1/4 cup fine almond flour
- 1 tsp. dried dill
- 1 tsp. dried chives
- 1 tsp. onion powder
- 1/2 tsp. garlic powder
- salt, to taste
- pepper, to taste

Instructions:

1. On a large plate or tray, combine dill, almond flour, and spices. Mix until well combined.
2. Dredge each fillet one at a time into the flour mix. Turn the fillet around until fully coated, and then transfer to a clean plate or tray. This may be refrigerated until ready to cook.
3. Place a large pan over medium-high heat.
4. Combine halves of butter and lemon juice. Swirl the pan to mix, lift occasionally to avoid burning the butter.
5. Allow the fish to cook for about 3 minutes.

6. Let the fish absorb all the lemony-butter mixture. Cook on low heat to avoid drying out the pan.
7. Add the remaining lemon juice and butter to the pan.
8. Turn the fish to cook the other side for 3 minutes more. Swirl around the pan to fully coat it with the juice.
9. Wait until it turns golden brown and the fish is cooked through.
10. Serve with buttered vegetables.

Salad Medley

Ingredients:

- 4 artichokes, halved
- 1/2 avocado, sliced into thin wedges
- 1/2 red, yellow, or green bell pepper, thinly sliced
- 1/4 squash, thinly sliced
- 1/2 zucchini, thinly sliced
- 1/2 red, yellow, or green onion, thinly sliced
- 1 cup mushrooms, thinly sliced
- 1 cup broccoli
- 1/4 cup broccoli sprouts
- 1 cup cauliflower
- 1 cup spinach
- 1 cup kale
- 1 bunch leeks, chopped
- 1/4 cup raw sunflower seeds, sprouted
- 1/4 cup raw almonds, sprouted
- 1/4 cup garbanzo beans, sprouted
- 1/4 cup mung beans, sprouted
- 1/4 cup red or green lentils, sprouted
- 1/4 cup purple cabbage, shredded
- 2 tbsp. extra-virgin olive oil

Instructions:

1. Steam vegetables in a saucepan with 1-inch water for 5 to 10 minutes.

2. Transfer steamed vegetables into a serving bowl.
3. Drizzle with extra-virgin olive oil.
4. Toss the vegetables.
5. Serve immediately.

Conclusion

Thank you again for getting this guide.

If you found this guide helpful, please take the time to share your thoughts and post a review. It'd be greatly appreciated!

Thank you and good luck!

References and Helpful Links

Palmer, Kelly. "Prediabetes: The 84 Million-Person Health Risk." The University of Arizona Health Sciences. August 6, 2019. https://uahs.arizona.edu/blog/2019-08-06/prediabetes-84-million-person-health-risk (accessed August 6, 2021).

Pritchard, Emma. "What is Insulin Resistance and Why Should You Care About It." Women's Health. February 21, 2019. https://www.womenshealthmag.com/uk/health/conditions/a26435775/insulin-resistance/ (accessed August 7, 2021).

"PCOS (Polycystic Ovary Syndrome) and Diabetes." Centers for Disease Control and Prevention. June 22, 2021. https://www.cdc.gov/diabetes/index.html (accessed August 8, 2021).

"Insulin Resistance & Prediabetes." National Institute of Diabetes and Digestive and Kidney Diseases. May 2018. https://www.niddk.nih.gov/health-information/diabetes/overview/what-is-diabetes/prediabetes-insulin-resistance (accessed August 8, 2021).

www.ingramcontent.com/pod-product-compliance
Lightning Source LLC
LaVergne TN
LVHW010438070526
838199LV00066B/6065